TRAUMATIC B

MW00913154

Cause, Consequence, and Challenge

Third Edition

Dennis P. Swiercinsky
Terrie L. Price
Leif Eric Leaf

Third Edition Revision by Terrie L. Price

All proceeds from the sale of this book support the
Brain Injury Association of Kansas & Greater Kansas City, Inc.
6405 Metcalf Ave., Suite 302
Telephone: (913) 754-8883
or (800) 783-1356

www.biaks.org

Published and distributed by
The Brain Injury Association of Kansas & Greater Kansas City, Inc.

Library of Congress Control Number: 2009910450

ISBN: 1-4392-6061-3

ACKNOWLEDGMENTS

The message herein has been written, mulled over, rewritten, reorganized, reflected upon, challenged, and rewritten again.... We hope it conveys the essence of compassion, knowledge, and quest that all who read this share in our lives with brain injury. Terrie, Leif, and I put together the initial draft. Through the carefully considered contributions of Mary Pat Beals, Elender Hill, and Marilyn Lawrenz, successive drafts were written. Jonathan Nye provided the illustrations. The technical editing of Jane Guthrie supplied the final polish to the text. Thank you all. Toward a unity of our essence, this work is dedicated to the person who grows from a brain injury.

D.P.S.
Kansas City, Missouri
January, 1987

The Revised Edition of this book includes added content that expands on several topics. Also, reference materials in the appendices have been added at the suggestion of several readers. Changes in wording made for the previous printing have been preserved. The goal to keep this book short, usable, and contemplative is still preserved. From its inception in 1986 to the additions in 1993, we hope the now more than 50,000 copies of this book are helping individuals and families accept the challenge of brain injury.

D.P.S.
Kansas City, Missouri
June, 1993

ILLUSTRATIONS

Illustrations provided by Jonathan Nye.

Left Lateral View of Whole Human Brain ... vi

Major Lobes of the Brain Cerebrum ... 14

Comparison of Normal and Damaged Cerebral Neurons ... 16

CONTENTS

ACKNOWLEDGMENTS ... iii

ILLUSTRATIONS ... iv

PREFACE TO THE THIRD EDITION ... 1

CAUSE

Chapter One
THE BRAIN INJURY EXPERIENCE ... 5

Chapter Two
SIMILARITIES AND DIFFERENCES AMONG PERSONS
WITH BRAIN INJURY... 9

CONSEQUENCE

Chapter Three
TYPES AND CONSEQUENCES OF BRAIN INJURY ... 13

Chapter Four
THE NEUROPSYCHOLOGICAL ASSESSMENT
AND REHABILITATION ... 27

CHALLENGE

Chapter Five
RECOVERY AND REHABILITATION ... 35

Chapter Six
ACCEPTING AND COPING WITH CHANGE ... 43

Chapter Seven
MANAGEMENT GUIDELINES ... 47

Chapter Eight
RESOURCES ... 51

GLOSSARIES ... 59
      Hospital Equipment
      Medications
      Neurological Tests and Procedures
      Neuropsychological Terms

APPENDICES ... 65
      Glasgow Coma Scale
      Revised Rancho Los Amigos Scale

ABOUT THE AUTHORS ... 69

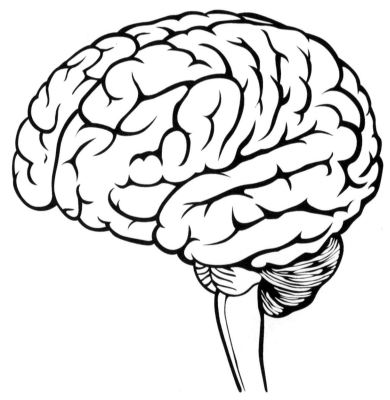

PREFACE TO THE THIRD EDITION

The "Red Book" was first published at the beginning of a period of intense research and education on the effects of traumatic brain injury and advocacy for survivors. In response, there was a tremendous increase in the number of medical rehabilitation programs opened and expanded throughout the nation. The National Head Injury Foundation, founded in 1980 by the mother of a child with a brain injury, saw exponential growth in members and the development of programs to meet their needs. Members not only included individuals with brain injuries and their families but also professional providers of medical and vocational services. Rehabilitation treatment centers and hospitals also joined the movement, all for the advancement of our growing knowledge of the major impact of brain injury and the critical importance of effective and timely treatment. Local, state, and federal resources became available for ongoing lifetime support.

Considerable growth has occurred since those early years. The National Head Injury Foundation is now the Brain Injury Association of America, a powerful advocacy group true to a mission of prevention, education, and resource building. Just as the national BIA was originally founded by the family member of an individual with a brain injury, state affiliates were opened and expanded through the diligent work of individuals with brain injury and their family members, in alliance with professional groups and organizations involved in treatment. The Brain injury Association of Kansas and Kansas City (BIAKS) was launched in 1982 through the leadership of Mary Pat Beals, the sister of a young woman who had sustained a traumatic brain injury in a motor vehicle crash.

The increasing awareness, education, and research in the field led to many critical advancements, such as the development of treatment standards by CARF (Commission on the Accreditation of Rehabilitation Facilities) and JCAHO (Joint Commission on the Accreditation

1

of Hospital Facilities), regulatory bodies in medical rehabilitation and hospital based brain injury care, ensuring standards of care for brain injury from emergency department through inpatient and outpatient rehabilitation, vocational training, and educational placement.

In 1997, IDEA (Individuals with Disabilities Education Act) was signed into law, including brain injury as a disability group requiring accommodations and special educational services. Research in brain injury has steadily increased and improved. Scientific studies support the effectiveness of treatment and the positive long-range outcomes that follow. Various states now have Medicaid brain injury waiver programs providing services that support individuals with brain injuries to be as maximally independent in their communities as possible. Programs have emerged across the country providing resources to public schools in educating teachers, counselors, and administrators on the educational needs of children with brain injuries. State vocational rehabilitation programs recognize brain injury as a unique disability category and many states require their vocational counselors to have training in brain injury, with the aim of achieving better vocational placement success. Disability groups share resources so that advancement of services and rights to one disability group often leads to benefits across several disability groups. The Americans with Disabilities Act (ADA) is one of many examples. Increased access to public facilities and transportation is a public benefit to everyone. The Internet now allows access to a body of information beyond our imagination thirty years ago, providing basic medical facts, statistics, resources, independent living aides, employment, and social networking. Professional specialization in brain injury rehabilitation is now an expectation for those who provide services to individuals with brain injury. Many fellowships are available to new neuropsychologists whereas there was a paucity of formal training programs when this book was first written.

Over the past thirty years, and even today, the thirst for information, services, and resources remains undiminished because the effects of brain injury can be monumental. This little book, dubbed "The Red Book," with thousands of copies printed to date, has provided key information and direction for brain injury survivors and their families. The lead author, Dennis Swiercinsky, PhD, ABN, began his career in neuropsychology by establishing the first set of published norms guiding neuropsychologists in the interpretation of test findings. Dennis was instrumental, along with Mary Pat, in the formative development of BIAKS. Their collaborative work and experience is well represented in the information and compassion provided in the Red Book.

Since its initial publication, the Red Book has earned validation through individuals with brain injuries and their family members, caregivers and providers. As a contributing author, I continue to receive comments from readers mostly that they felt like someone really understood their experience. Medical and rehabilitation providers new to the field have commented that the book provides a basic and useful review of the nature and effects of brain injury.

The advancements in research and education demand a periodic review and update on informational material. The challenge for updating the Red Book is to concisely include new knowledge and to retain the original impact. We have opted to retain the Red Book material with few changes to the original writing. We have substituted the current language of "brain injury" for the terms "head injury" and "traumatic head injury" in order to be consistent with more recent common terminology. Some chapters now begin with new content addressing some additional information and considerations.

As I reflect on the writings of the original Red Book, I am reminded of a major change. When the Red Book was first written, the majority of survivors of brain injury experienced moderate to severe brain injury. Advancements in treatment, prevention and safety have lead to a decrease in moderate to severe brain injuries. It is now recognized that people experiencing concussion and mild brain injury are just as much in need of information and support. While many of the effects of severe to mild brain injury are similar, there are major differences. The introductory chapters herein will provide a perspective in this regard.

I close this preface to the Third Edition with gratitude to Dennis for his leadership, to Mary Pat for her tenacity and drive, to BIAKS for ongoing advocacy, and to the many individuals who live with brain injury, and their families or caregivers, for their shared experience that keeps us centered on the message of hope, courage and hard work.

Terrie Price, Ph.D., ABPP
June, 2010

Chapter One

THE BRAIN INJURY EXPERIENCE

Half a million Americans experience severe brain injury each year. Most of these individuals survive, largely a credit to remarkable advances in emergency medical care. Those who have defied death, however, begin a journey of rehabilitation that is challenging and just as remarkable. Some will return to their previous style of living; some will undergo lengthy rehabilitation; some will cope with changes that will permanently alter their previous life-style. Brain injury raises many questions: What has happened? What can be expected for recovery? What will the injury mean for the rest of the person's and his or her family's lives? This book provides information and understanding for patients and families who likely will live with the specter of brain injury for years and maybe forever.

A traumatic brain injury occurs when the skull slams against a windshield, the ground, or some other stationary object. The compression, twisting, and distortion of the brain inside the skull associated with this impact causes localized as well as widespread damage throughout the brain. Usually a period of unconsciousness immediately follows the trauma. In a severe brain injury, this may last from minutes to weeks or even months. The individual never remembers the injury, the time immediately prior to it, or the several hours, sometimes days or weeks, that follow. This occurs because of direct damage to the brain tissue that controls learning and new memory. Damage to the brain may continue after the impact if bleeding occurs, breathing stops, or the brain tissue swells.

In a minor traumatic brain injury there may be no loss of consciousness, but only a dazed feeling for a while, possibly followed by head-ache, drowsiness, or other unusual feelings. The potential for having sustained minor brain injury, though, is present. Although

5

acute medical care may be minimal and recovery rapid, families of persons sustaining mild brain injury should still be sensitive to subtle cognitive and personality changes from normal, preinjury behavior.

Brain injury can occur for other reasons as well. Near drowning, heart attacks, lung problems, chemical and drug reactions, and infections may cause inadequate blood flow to the brain, resulting in some brain cell death. These cases produce behavior and adjustment problems similar to those seen in traumatic brain injury, even though the mechanism of damage is different.

The vulnerability of the brain to damage is rather alarming. Despite its being encased in the thick bone of the skull, even minor trauma can injure delicate brain tissue. The fact that the brain is responsible for virtually everything we do, feel, learn, and experience makes any amount of injury a disturbance that can produce lifestyle consequences.

After the life has been saved, the individual medically stabilized and perhaps even home, and some sense of day-to-day balance regained, the meaning of "brain injury" becomes starkly apparent. Although relatively rapid rehabilitation progress is usually seen early on—learning to walk and talk again, learning self-care, regaining physical strength—a disturbing change in the person who has experienced a severe brain injury may persist. Families may be jolted by the realization that their family member that has sustained a brain injury is now a "new" person, with immense, immediate, and complex needs.

The key to healthy adjustment to any degree of brain injury is to become sensitive to the enduring changes caused by the injury. Learning to understand and take control of those changes instead of succumbing to them can mean the difference between a future of happiness or a future of grief. All but the mildest brain injury produces lasting differences in how one thinks, feels, and experiences life.

The multiple effects of trauma and the therapy needs of the person with a brain injury are varied. There is one effect, however, that is universal. Called "shearing stress lesions" or "diffuse axonal injury," some brain cells are permanently torn apart one from another at the moment of the injurious impact. Although many of these cells do not die, they are never again connected to one another in the same way. Regardless of possible complications, such as skull fracture, hematoma, swelling, infection, or blood vessel tears, the effects of shearing stress lesions persist. It is this type of lesion that causes lingering memory and learning difficulties, occasional confusion, concrete as opposed to abstract thinking, and subtle personality changes that are ever present yet elusive and difficult to understand.

As with any major life event, severe brain injury changes the individual and his or her family forever. Experiencing a potentially life-threatening situation, followed by intensive medical care, long-term rehabilitation, the loneliness and fear that accompanies the unknown, the waiting, the constant reassessment of personal values and goals, the guilt that follows denial, the joys and tears of helping and being helped, coping with changed plans, the struggle to make realistic plans, the excitement of change, the breakthroughs in mental and cognitive recovery—all accompany the experience known as brain injury. It is dynamic and lasts at least years, and often a lifetime.

Throughout the long process of adjusting and coping, persons with brain injury and their family members are faced with learning something about brain-behavior relationships. Distinguishing between behavior caused by brain injury and that which is a product of native personality often baffles families. Knowing what to do next to cope with subtle, sometimes intensely perplexing, life-planning questions confronts persons who are brain injured, their families, and rehabilitation providers. To seek understanding of the complex brain is an important beginning in reducing the anxiety and frustration of the brain injury experience. Knowledge of what has happened and is happening inside the brain and about the psychological and emotional process of recovery helps provide a sense of control over the chaos, making hope seem realistic.

The haunting questions—Will the person who has been injured ever be normal again? Will he or she make a full recovery? Is it reasonable to hope that the survivor of brain injury will get better? Will we ever get used to this new person?—are not easily answered. In fact, "coming to terms" with these questions is the essence of the psychological aspect of rehabilitation. Facing reality with a new sense of values is necessary. "Normality," or the idealized memory of normalcy, can no longer be idolized. "Recovery" takes on new meaning including how to do and think in different ways. "Hope" becomes an attitude of active conquest, not of passive waiting. The "new person" is a mix of the former personality and the courageous accomplishments of facing a challenge without retreat.

Called the "Silent Epidemic," brain injury is the most common cause of death or disability today for people under age 40. According to the Centers of Disease Control (CDC) and Prevention, at least 1.7 million people sustain a traumatic brain injury every year in the United States. The number of people with TBI who are not seen in a hospital or emergency department or who receive no care is currently unknown. Ninety-eight percent of these people will live and want to lead as normal lives as possible. The sense of helplessness and powerlessness that initially overcomes a person who has sustained a brain injury and his or her family can be reduced and even conquered as knowledge replaces ignorance, hope replaces hopelessness, and courage replaces fear.

Chapter Two

SIMILARITIES AND DIFFERENCES AMONG PERSONS WITH BRAIN INJURY

Like anyone who acquires a label, "brain-injured persons" are still whole, *unique people*. Use of the term "brain-injured" when referring to a person is a disservice; the label preempts the uniqueness and conjures a stereotype. Putting the person first, as in "a person who has had a brain injury," preserves respect for individuality and diminishes the chance of knowing that person only in terms of some expectation of disability.

Depending on the severity and location of brain injury, the possible complications, the age of the person, current and former health status, and preexisting intellectual and personality characteristics, the outcome of brain injury will be different. Some persons who experience brain injury will be unconscious a few minutes, some will be in a coma for weeks. Some will "wake up" very gradually over the course of days, others will seem to have regained normal arousal almost instantly. Sometimes there will be a veil of confusion, of being "not with it," of a "distance" that will persist and vary for weeks or months. In addition to cognitive (thinking) changes, the injured person may show self-centeredness, a lack of affectionate responsiveness, and a lack of depth to the personality. These changes are often disturbing to families, who realize their loved one is no longer the same, and who do not understand the change. Whereas some patients will eventually recover with almost no noticeable problems, others may require a great deal of personal care for the rest of their lives.

Nearly all persons who sustain a brain injury experience damage to the axis or base of the brain, known as the *brain stem*, which affects heart rate, breathing, blood pressure, body temperature, and other vital functions. Although these functions usually recover and stabilize soon after injury, other functions of the brain stem seem not to recover as well: those of attention span and short-term immediate memory. Individual reactions to new difficulties in remembering or paying attention to everyday details depend on how the individual may have reacted to similar but less severe problems before the injury. Factors such as the extent of injury, preexisting style of coping with frustration, attitude toward the injury, family support, rigidity or flexibility in personal adjustment, and attitudes toward life itself also affect such reactions.

Over time, often years, the individual develops new personality traits, regaining and sharpening some of his or her preexisting characteristics and acquiring new ones. The individual also learns, with arduous persistence, new skills and can often return to work or school. Or, if not, he or she can assume a meaningful life in other ways. All of this depends on the physical consequences of the injury as well as on the personal commitment to rehabilitation, constant family participation and support, acceptance of new ideas and change, and the willingness to do things differently to function more efficiently.

It is important to keep a perspective about the changes a brain injury brings. Everyone is disabled in some respect, but we normally focus on our strengths and potentials. This is also the focus in rehabilitation, sharpening residual skills and learning new ones. There is a prideful feeling that can accompany being different, unique, something more than mere normal. There is a limiting feeling about being disabled, something second class.

Despite the oftentimes catastrophic results of brain injury, learning how to erase or at least minimize its disabling consequences is the real challenge. Doing, thinking, and saying whatever is necessary to see yourself as different yet respectfully unique is the challenge in the face of loss and disappointment. Life change that comes suddenly can result in a de-powering feeling because it is so overwhelming. Building a perspective of pride, of making being different being good, or at least okay, represents healthy growth and positive psychological adjustment.

A fallacy of any illness or injury is in comparing present functioning with what was. Most people experience at least some periods of dissatisfaction with the quality of life. If this becomes a severe preoccupation, it may lead to depression or even to suicide. This imbalance created in the failure to accept the unchangeable and to change what one can defeats rehabilitation. Quality of life is defined in one's own terms, but often outside help is valuable in developing a positive, self-accepting attitude.

The question often asked about a person with a brain injury is, "Will he (or she) ever be the same again?" This question often reflects sadness and grief that the injured individual may be "lost" forever. Actually, from day to day none of us are ever the same again. A brain injury produces brain tissue change: some lost cells, some disconnected cells, some cells that have "healed" but with different connections than before. The physical and emotional experience of the injury, intensive medical care, the process of rehabilitation, and time itself change one forever. There may be at least the threads of the familiar personality, interests, and characteristics, but everyone involved must adapt to a new uniqueness, a personality molded from the past, the physical and emotional effects of trauma, and a new view to the future.

It is fallacious and defeating to wait for the old person to come back after a brain injury. No, the person who has had a brain injury will never be the same again. But after the loss of the familiar person is mourned and the dramatic upheaval of changes settles down, the challenge of living begins anew.

"Recovery" from brain injury means "growing" from brain injury: restoring cognitive abilities where possible, accepting new ways of doing things, changing career or life plans. This change process is really life long, with periods of accelerated growth and periods of plateau during which little seems to be happening. Recovery from brain injury, in this sense, never stops. As humans, we are always striving—for better self-acceptance, more learning, and greater happiness and satisfaction.

The more we learn about brain injury and the functioning of the brain, the more we come to respect individuality. Modern neuroscience is complex. Current theories of brain functioning are fashioned after complex mathematical models of how billions of neurons work together in systems of neural networks. Even the most formidable of these theories actually accounts for a large measure of unpredictability. Only *ranges* of outcomes from the models are possible. One neuroscientist likens fickle brain functioning to the weather, more than to a computer.

The similarities among the effects of brain injury are fairly universal: memory changes, thinking style changes, emotional changes. But, underlying these similarities are the differences of the individual personalities. Uniqueness gives us each a sense of importance. The common effects of brain injury only force upon us the need to confront our new uniqueness. While this is usually unsettling at first, it becomes the enduring challenge.

Chapter Three

TYPES AND CONSEQUENCES OF BRAIN INJURY

With hope and a commitment to understand the intense experience of brain injury, knowledge is the greatest weapon against fear, misunderstanding, and helplessness. This chapter offers a brief journey through neuroscience, describing the physical and behavioral characteristics brought about by brain injury. No individual will experience all of these changes, but many, particularly the cognitive and personality characteristics, will emerge in some fashion and to some extent throughout the rehabilitation phase.

The Brain

The brain controls virtually all of the body's functions, from the vital processes of breathing to sensing and moving, from the highest centers of thinking and judgment to the emotional reactions to it all. Understanding what happens to the brain in brain injury requires a fundamental appreciation of its structure.

The **brain stem** connects the brain with the spinal cord. The **reticular formation** and other structures of the brain stem control consciousness, arousal, and vital functions such as breathing, respiration, and pulse rate. All information from the body from the neck down passes through the brain stem on its way to being processed in higher brain regions. Similarly, all directives from the brain for body activity must pass through the brain stem on their way to the muscles and bodily organs. Unfortunately, the brain stem sits at the base of the brain, near bony areas, in a vulnerable position that is easily damaged during trauma. **Cranial nerves**, positioned near the brain stem, are also sometimes damaged, causing dysfunction to eye muscles, facial and voice control, muscles involved in swallowing, hearing, and smell.

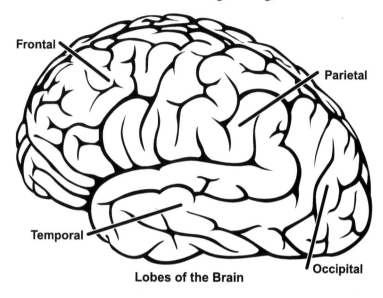

Frontal

Parietal

Temporal

Occipital

Lobes of the Brain

Fig. 1. Lateral view of the cerebral cortex.

The **cerebellum** lies in twin cupped areas of the cranium just behind and slightly above the brain stem. Responsible mostly for coordinating movement and remembering habitual movement patterns, the cerebellum is sometimes damaged but often not severely; it is relatively well protected, compared to many other areas of the brain.

The **cerebrum** is the major part of the brain, in which virtually all "higher" brain activity takes place: language, thinking, initiation of activity, emotional control, creativity, remembering, learning, mathematical reasoning, and expression of personality. The covering of the cerebrum, the **cortex**, is where these activities take place. The nerve cells beneath the cortex are mostly tracts of nerve fibers that provide intracerebral communication. Because the cells of the cortex lie at the surface of the brain, they are susceptible to damage when the cerebrum slams into the inside of the cranium (skull) during a trauma. Some systems of nerve tracts (the **limbic system**, for example, which helps control memory and emotions) are vulnerable to damage by virtue of their extensive representation throughout the brain. **Ventricles**, pools within the brain, contain fluid; these sometimes fill excessively and cause pressure damage to the rest of the cerebral structures.

Each right and left half, or **hemisphere**, of the cerebrum is divided into four areas or lobes, each corresponding to a more-or-less distinct area of the cortex and each representing more-or-less specific functions.

The **frontal lobe** is the emotional control center and highest intellective area of the brain. It is almost always injured somewhat by being situated at the front of the brain and getting slammed into the front of the cranium. The frontal lobe is involved in a variety of cognitive functions, including language, creative thought, problem solving, initiation of movement, judgment, and impulse control. It is also involved in self-awareness and self-monitoring of socially appropriate behaviors.

The **parietal lobes** lying at the top midsection of each hemisphere are involved in sensation, reading, listening, awareness of spatial relationships, and memory. The parietal lobes provide the site for most basic intellectual abilities, such as the "3-Rs" of reading, writing, and arithmetic.

Localized laterally along both of the hemispheres are the **temporal lobes**. These areas, like the frontal lobes, are especially vulnerable to damage as they are hurled against the sides of the bony pockets that contain them. Memory, language, sequencing, and musical ability are some of the functions of the temporal lobes.

The **occipital lobes** are found at the very back of the brain and are the primary sites of visual perception. Of the four lobes in each hemisphere, the occipital is usually least damaged in trauma. However, very subtle changes in how efficiently the occipital lobes work in carrying out visual perception is often seen. This is because the visual tracts must pass all the way from the eyes, through the frontal and temporal lobes before they get to the occipital lobes. Damage to the tracts anywhere along the way, or injury to the occipital cortex itself, can cause sometimes subtle disruption in seeing and perception.

The Physical Damage

Structural and physiological damage always occurs as a result of brain injury. The type and location of damage is the product of multiple factors including the mechanism of injury, physiological reaction, and subsequent complications that might occur. Preexisting conditions such as alcohol use, drugs, certain diseases, and prior brain injury also may affect the degree of injury as well as recovery potential.

The most common type of brain injury is the **closed head injury**. When the head collides with another surface, damage is caused to the brain as it is hurled against the inside of the skull. The blow may fracture the cranium, injure the scalp, and cause intracranial complications such as blood clots and blocked ventricles or blood vessels.

When an object such as a bullet pierces the skull and causes brain injury, the result is known as a **penetrating** (or open) **head injury**. Whereas closed head injury often occurs when the skull moves rapidly into an object, penetrating head injury usually occurs when another object breaks through the skull with powerful force. Sometimes in an impact injury a portion of the skull is broken and pushed into the brain, whereby the brain sustains overall shearing stress lesions (discussed in Chapter One) as well as the localized skull penetration injury. Penetrating injury adds significant complications, such as potential for infection and focal death of brain cells.

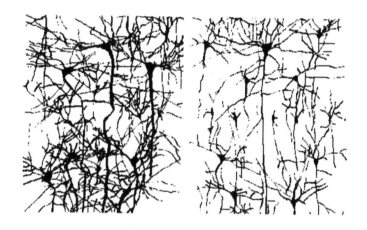

Fig. 2. Effects of trauma: Before and after injury.

Closed or penetrating head injury refers to physical trauma of sufficient magnitude to cause injury to living tissue, beginning with injury to soft tissue of the skin and muscles. The greater the force of the injury, the more the effect of the force travels through the soft tissue into the bony skull and on into the brain tissue.

Contusions and hematomas are two common forms of **focal lesions** caused by concussion. A **contusion** is a bruise of a specific area of the brain. In closed head injury, this usually occurs in the brain stem, frontal lobes, and temporal lobes. Small blood vessels break, and the surrounding tissue is deprived of normal blood flow. **Anoxia**, lack of oxygen due to interruption of the supply of fresh blood, may cause brain cell death. A **hematoma** is a contusion on a larger scale. When larger blood vessels tear, blood may flow freely (a **hemorrhage**) and form a pocket of blood large enough to press against adjoining tissue and cause pressure damage in addition to the damage caused by insufficient flow of blood to the intended brain tissue. Any disruption in blood supply to neural tissue is called **ischemia**, and often causes **necrosis** (death) of the deprived tissue.

In all forms of brain injury, shearing stress lesions, discussed in Chapter One, are caused by major concussive force. These result in **diffuse axonal injury**, where the nerve cells are torn apart one from another. Cell death usually does not occur, but the normal transmission of nerve impulses necessary for efficient thinking, memory, and self-monitoring of behavior is disrupted. Neurochemical changes usually take place as well, further reducing the efficiency of brain cell functioning.

In addition to diffuse axonal injury, concussion may produce other effects of contusion including brain swelling, sudden electrochemical changes and brain chemical toxicity, hematoma, skull fracture, and other injuries. Concussion is usually rated mild to severe. In very mild concussion, the individual does not lose consciousness but may still sustain some brain injury, although usually temporary. In more severe concussion, loss of consciousness occurs as a result of brain stem trauma. If the force of the concussion is severe enough to cause more than a brief disruption of brain stem neurochemical activity and normal nerve tissue structure, the individual usually lapses into a coma (profound unconsciousness). A coma indicates severe and serious damage.

The mechanism of coma is not well understood but involves a major shutting down of brain functioning. If damage is done to life-sustaining centers of the brain, the individual may need to be placed on life-support such as mechanical ventilation (breathing) until the brain tissue heals sufficiently and coma begins to resolve.

A coma always produces **amnesia**. Inability to remember what happened for a period of time before an injury is called **retrograde**

amnesia. It may extend back in time minutes to days before the injury and is never completely recoverable. **Post-traumatic amnesia** is the period following the injury in which memory cannot be established in the brain. This problem gradually resolves after a few weeks or months. But, because of the sudden impact to the memory creating centers of the brain, the ability to recall the actual event of the trauma is almost never possible.

When concussion occurs, the body's physiology triggers a reaction which sends more blood to the injured area. Normally, this is desirable because greater than normal blood flow helps fight infection and aids the recovery of damaged tissue. In the brain, however, this reaction can be lethal. As the brain can expand in response to this **swelling** only so much, the added pressure on tissue can cause further damage. Cerebrospinal fluid flow is also interrupted and can cause additional pressure damage to nerve cells as ventricles fill beyond their normal capacity.

If swelling occurs, eventually additional fluids will accumulate in the brain as a result of the contusion-reaction gone awry. This causes a condition known as **edema**. Swelling and edema require immediate medical attention or the individual will die, or at least sustain even more brain injury.

Depending on conditions that no one fully understands, **seizures** may occur following brain injury, sometimes starting months later ("late-onset" seizures). Essentially, these are caused by impaired electrochemical activity in damaged tissue. Scar tissue development may initiate seizures. A seizure can range from a brief interruption in conscious awareness to grand mal tonic-clonic rhythmic contractions of the whole body. Because there is potential for seizures to occur, medications are often administered as a preventative for several months or years following a brain injury. Although the precise reason for post-traumatic seizures is unknown, they are usually effectively controlled with medications. (Sometimes excessive stress or alcohol consumption can start a seizure in a person who has had a brain injury. Use of alcohol is strongly discouraged for anyone who is at risk for seizure. Similarly, avoidance of a stressful lifestyle is also recommended.)

Brain injury is a dynamic condition. Torn axons, swelling, and contusion will produce a natural reaction of living tissue to recover. If damage is severe enough, however, the immediate recovery reaction can produce temporary chaos. New nerve cells are called into action to try to take over for damaged ones; neurochemical and vascular changes may excite some areas of the brain and inhibit others. Out of the chaos, however, and usually with critical help from doctors, the body and brain immediately start a process to recover biological balance, the process known as **homeostasis**.

The mechanisms of brain injury, let alone normal brain functioning, are indeed complex. Physical, electrical, and chemical disruptions occur. Different behavioral reactions, from lethargy to combativeness, are observed following coma recovery, depending on multiple damage and physiological factors. Immediate medical attention is necessary to save the life; constant and long-term psychological and rehabilitative vigilance is necessary to mend and gradually mold the expression of life back into its most meaningful and productive form.

Once the individual has recovered from coma and is beginning to exhibit awareness of surroundings and other people, the focus of doctors and family usually shifts from the physical to the behavioral and cognitive problems. Medical stability requires intense and careful effort and immediate worries center around the life-threatening injuries. When such worries are no longer an issue, observation and treatment of the behavioral, cognitive, and psychological changes exhibited by the injured person take precedence.

The Behavioral, Cognitive, and Psychological Changes

As noted previously the behavioral, cognitive (thinking), and psychological (personality and emotional) changes that occur as a result of brain injury vary for each individual and are partially dependent on pre-injury personality, psychological adjustment, intelligence, and learning style. The characteristics described here are common with brain injury, but not universal among all persons.

Among the many potential cognitive and psychological changes, memory, attention, and personality are almost universally described by families as problems. As these are very complex brain functions, it is important to realize that the injured person is not being intentionally obstinate when he or she forgets something or behaves childishly. Rehabilitation is aimed at transforming these changes so they are as limiting as possible.

Motor Problems. Motor problems can be quite varied, involving injuries to the complex motor (movement) systems of the brain, spinal cord, and peripheral (non-brain) nerves. **Hemiparesis** is a paralysis (lack of movement) of one side of the body; **quadriparesis** involves both legs and both arms. Other movement problems may include poor balance, difficulty planning and carrying out movements (**apraxia**), poor coordination (**ataxia**), or unstable muscle tone (**spasticity**). Combativeness and restlessness are exhibited by many persons with brain injury early after the trauma, when the brain is incapable of an orderly control of movements and intentions. **Vestibular** (balance) problems result from heightened sensitivity to movement, and **proprioceptive** (movement feedback) problems result from deficits in feedback from the muscles to the brain. Concurrent with brain injury, the person may have sustained damage to muscles and joints (orthopedic deficits), causing similarly appearing problems.

Residual motor problems are almost always a permanent consequence of major or minor brain injury. Even subtle compromise in fine motor dexterity may make using a keyboard or manipulating very small objects difficult. These factors must be taken into account in long-range vocational planning following a brain injury.

Perceptual Problems. The sensory systems (touch, vision, smell, hearing, taste) are as complex as motor systems. Brain injury may cause a variety of changes to any of the senses. **Hemiesthesia** is the loss of touch sensation (including pain and pressure) on one side of the body. Heightened sensitivity to touch results in a phenomenon known as **tactile defensiveness.** Loss of ability to see things on one side of the visual field (hemianopsia, or **visual field deficit**), neglect or ignoring things on one side of the body (**unilateral neglect**), double vision (**diplopia**), or problems in depth perception and visual acuity may affect the visual sense. Changes in auditory (hearing), olfactory (smell), or gustatory (taste) senses may occur as well. The nerves responsible for smell and taste are particularly vulnerable to damage during trauma because they lie underneath the frontal lobes, and many persons who have had a brain injury report reduced acuity or loss of these senses.

Speech Problems. Difficulty understanding information (**receptive aphasia**) or expressing thoughts through speech or writing (**expressive aphasia**) results from complex injuries to large key brain areas, usually located in the left hemisphere. Such problems are usually accompanied by cognitive problems as well. **Dysarthria** refers to difficulty pronouncing or articulating words or phrases, due to injured nerves that control the muscles involved in speech production. Volume limitations in speaking may result from subtle breathing problems and injuries to the nerves of the vocal cords.

The general area of complex **cognitive communications** refers to the thinking aspect of speaking and listening. Brain injury affects how easily a person can find the words to express a thought or to formulate sequences of words to convey intended meaning. Subtle residual hesitations, longer time needed to get a point across, or occasional confusion in understanding the spoken intentions of others often follows brain injury.

Coping with and adapting to these changes means that the person must give himself or herself more time and patience in communicating with others. Use of written instead of verbal communication may allow more time for thoughtful composition and organization of thoughts. As with any area of change brought about because of brain injury, creative adjustment and adaptation always challenges the person who has had a brain injury.

Regulatory Problems. Becoming easily fatigued is one of the most common regulatory problems reported by the person who has had a brain injury, especially relatively soon after injury. This situation usually improves during rehabilitation, but shorter work periods may always be needed. Brain injury also may produce changes in the body's ability to regulate sleep, temperature, and food and liquid consumption. Change in the ability to sense the need to empty one's bowels or bladder may require special attention to strict habits. Sexual arousal may be greatly reduced or increased after damage to specific deep areas of the brain. Acne, sweating, and other physical disturbances may occur due to disruption in the brain's control mechanisms.

Susceptibility to overload and stress is almost always seen, at least early on, as a consequence of brain injury. Sometimes this is easily observed in that the individual cannot seem to take much stimulation—too many people, colors, shapes, sounds, and things going on at the same time. Returning to school or work too soon may reveal this problem, not only in being unable to keep up with former demands but in experiencing stress with too much happening at once. Of course, this problem emerges in busy environments more than in calm ones. Being sensitive to the potential for subtle overload can help prevent such problems.

Cognitive and Personality Problems. Cognitive, or intellectual-type, difficulties and personality changes resulting from brain injury seem to linger and be more problematic over time than do the previously described problems. We seem to have more difficulty accepting or adjusting to problems that cause us to forget, not think too clearly sometimes, make rash or impulsive decisions, or even to have trouble making decisions at all.

Cognitive problems encompass an array of possibilities, including memory failures; difficulty or slowness in learning new information, performing arithmetical calculations, or being flexible in solving unique problems; getting lost even in familiar places; getting confused with directions or left-right orientation; and having trouble getting dressed (or doing any number of previously familiar things) because of the difficulty in following a routine or logical sequence of steps. The list may seem endless. Careful observation and neuropsychological assessment (discussed in the next chapter) will help define such problems and lead to an understanding of which therapy might help recover, or at least improve, these deficits.

It is relatively easy to understand the brain injury behind cognitive problems. But, understanding psychological problems as based in brain dysfunction and the brain's inefficiency due to injury requires more sensitivity. Both for the person who has experienced brain injury and for his or her family and friends, awareness of the basis of psychological problems can be the foundation for adaptation and improving functioning. The common, though variable, psychological consequences of brain injury that may persist for some time include the following:

Denial: In an effort to appear whole and unimpaired, an individual either denies that anything has changed or minimizes the recognition of change. Also, as some persons are truly unaware that they have changed and do not realize the existence of problems, unrealistic attitudes and/or excuses usually result.

Apathy: Actually a form of denial, the person with a brain injury may show little interest in anything. This reaction, in preventing any activity, often is used to protect oneself from failure. Reduced motivation can also be a direct result of damage to the frontal lobes.

Emotional Lability: Inappropriate and/or exaggerated laughing or crying due to a loss of emotional control may relate to a damaged limbic system or frontal lobes of the brain. Sometimes the individual will switch from "high" to "low" emotions unpredictably. Emotions may also be intense and quick to appear.

Impulsivity and Disinhibition: Characteristic impulsivity is observed when the individual acts or speaks without considering the consequences, attempts tasks beyond his or her capabilities, and starts tasks and answers questions before hearing full directions. Impulsivity and disinhibition are often linked to changes in attention span.

Frustration Intolerance: Giving up easily and an unwillingness to stick to tasks because they become so frustrating must be addressed early in rehabilitation. Failure to treat this problem will undermine overall efforts in cognitive rehabilitation; the individual will learn early on to give up or not attempt tasks at all to avoid frustration.

Lack of Insight: When the individual is unable to understand and integrate the facts of a situation, the resulting lack of insight may appear as blatant illogical arguing. This characteristic produces poor decision making in general. Ironically, once a decision is made, even new facts or information acquired do not easily produce a change in the original decision.

Inflexibility: Examples of this characteristic are seen in poor problem solving, due to failure to entertain alternative solutions, failure to evaluate possible influences of two or more variables, and inability to look at problems from someone else's perspective. Inflexibility is also seen in difficulty attending to or performing more than one thing at a time and using experience to cope with new problems.

Confusion: The injured brain processes less information than it used to, within a given amount of time. This, and a fluctuating attention span, contributes to the potential for confusion. A slower paced and simplified environment and taking more time to accomplish a learning task can help reduce confusion.

Forgetting: The number one symptom reported by persons who have sustained brain injury is a change in memory. Ability to grasp and remember things—facts, appointments, plans—exhibits varying degrees of unreliability. While techniques may be learned to improve short-term memory, damage to the limbic system is the primary cause of memory problems.

Verbosity: An apparent inability to control the amount of talking, sometimes rambling a great deal, usually reflects an ineffective attempt to gain attention, to appear intelligent, or merely to avoid the fear of feeling left out. Sometimes, rambling is due to the person just feeling like he or she is unable to organize thoughts sufficiently to make a point. This, as well as many other psychological consequences of brain injury, stems from a loss of sensitivity toward one's own behavior and social actions.

Perseveration: Related to verbosity is the tendency to repeat or focus on a topic excessively. Often the person does not recall having said something and repeats the same thing over and over.

Confabulation: Due to a combination of confusion, forgetfulness, and unwillingness to appear impaired, an individual may fabricate ideas that are partly or completely false. Bits and pieces of real or formerly understood information may be incorporated into a story that the person truly believes, being unaware of the inaccuracy. Sometimes confabulation masquerades as a tendency to be overly sure of something that everyone else knows is inaccurate.

Lack of Initiation and Follow-through: This inability to start actions independently of others and carry a sequence of steps through to completion is often corrected through close supervision and provision of structure.

Slow and Inefficient Thinking: Poor sequencing, erratic and unreliable memory, periodic confusion, and sensory overload all contribute to what appears to be, simply, inefficient thinking. Slowness to respond to others is characteristic as well.

Poor Judgment and Poor Reasoning: The individual may not always be able to analyze a situation correctly or take into account the probable consequences of actions. Difficulty drawing logical conclusions with analysis and support of facts is evident.

Social Imperception: Social skills are impaired when the individual lacks sensitivity and emotional concern about his or her surroundings and disregards usual priorities. As with most cognitive and personality changes following brain injury, the individual is usually unaware of the problem, which is due directly to the physiological injury to the brain. Rehabilitation is aimed at bringing about awareness of these problems and helping the individual make adjustment changes.

Observing the consequences of brain injury sometimes gives one the impression that the affected individual is demonstrating a developmental regression, as though he or she is a child again. Unfortunately, that childish behavior sometimes lingers and becomes very disruptive both to the family and to the patient's recovery. Rehabilitation focuses on every one of these issues and, within the limits of the brain and preexisting cognitive and personality resources, brings the person to his or her fullest possible functioning.

This chapter has described many of the consequences of brain injury. It is easy to think in terms of losses, inabilities, and deficits. The dramatic and sudden changes in functions following injury contrast with the level of functioning which characterized the individual prior to the injury. We must be careful to focus our attention on changes within our ability to *positively* influence these changes and not to succumb to them.

As the healing (both physiological and psychological) continues, the person with a brain injury must learn ways to improve memory, become more self-aware, regain self-respect and confidence, know limits and strengths, and strive for self-accepting adjustment. The consequences of brain injury are always a combination of physical injury *and attitude*. Time and a commitment to work on taking more control over the undesirable changes produced by injury contribute to rehabilitation outcome.

Respect for individual differences and a certain amount of unpredictability in brain injury recovery has been established. While several common themes of functional changes are observed in persons with brain injury, it is necessary to gain a comprehensive understanding of the impact of injury on an individual's lifestyle. Although most persons who sustain brain injury experience change in memory functions, the specific consequences for each individual's lifestyle and work potential must be assessed. The individual's strengths, learning style preferences, and other resources must be understood in order to appreciate how a functional change or limitation will be experienced or how it will need to be addressed in rehabilitation.

Chapter Four

THE NEUROPSYCHOLOGICAL ASSESSMENT AND REHABILITATION

Neuropsychology is the study of brain-behavior relationships, involving the assessment of cognitive functioning as well as emotional impact resulting from brain injury. The assessment process, as described in the following paragraphs, is varied according to the needed information and capacity of the individual to complete an assessment. During early hospitalization, the acute nature of the injury typically does not allow for more than an abbreviated screening of select cognitive functions indicative of basic cognitive integrity, mostly related to memory, attention, and language. As the individual improves, a more comprehensive assessment will evaluate cognitive and emotional areas in greater depth. This will include assessment of the complex nature of memory, attention, language, reasoning, initiation and planning, and cognitive processing speed.

Why complete a comprehensive neuropsychological evaluation? Sometimes, individuals mistakenly believe the assessment only addresses deficits, which typically raises anxiety. However, a thorough neuropsychological assessment also provides an assessment of strengths. The balanced information is applied in developing strategies to promote recovery, return to meaningful activities (as much as possible) such as driving, school, work, and independent living. For long-term success in reaching these goals, an individual needs to build on their strengths, and develop strategies to minimize impact of areas of difficulty. During recovery, knowledge of specific areas of difficulty guide treatment planning. For example, an assessment is used in identifying the necessary accommodations and modifications that may be needed in order to progress to greater independence. Such information, can guide in the identification of useful strategies that can be pursued in various therapies. For example, some individuals may not be as successful in using a planner/calendar book. But they maybe successful using timers and similar environmental cues as reminders. Adolescents and young adults are more inclined to successfully use electronic devices such as their phones, PDAs and computers rather than watches or traditional calendars. The opposite is more likely true among older and senior adults. The first steps in returning to independence are very different for an individual who has sustained a mild brain injury relative to the challenges faced in living with a moderate to severe brain injury.

The challenge of neuropsychological assessment is to develop a clear picture of an individual's strengths and weaknesses across a wide variety of cognitive and emotional functions in order that realistic rehabilitation planning can occur. A significant value of neuropsychological assessment includes evaluating improvement over the recovery period, which can be very rewarding and reassuring to the individual survivor and his or her family.

The neuropsychologist's involvement in an individual's care cannot be understated and extends well beyond assessment inclusive of providing continuing education on brain injury adaptation and recovery. Throughout their treatment course, neuropsychologists actively participate with the team in developing an individualized and timely treatment plan. Often times, the neuropsychologist is called in to provide education and training to teachers and vocational specialists involved in aiding the person in his or her return to activities.

A rehabilitation psychologist is a specialist within psychology that applies psychological (including neuropsychological) knowledge in helping individuals with disabilities and chronic health conditions in their welfare, community participation, and quality of life. Living with a brain injury can involve adjusting to changes in many areas of one's life. It is not uncommon for an individual living with a brain injury, or their family, to consult with a neuropsychologist or rehabilitation psychologist at different times in dealing with new challenges that continually emerge.

A clinical neuropsychological assessment provides a comprehensive and detailed description of the unique behavioral, cognitive, and psychological consequences of brain trauma. An assessment of this type documents the array of functional strengths and weaknesses so that rehabilitation can tap resources to help the individual adjust to or compensate for disabilities. The neuropsychologist uses scientific techniques to infer premorbid (preexisting) characteristics of the individual and to provide an index of the extent and type of changes brought about by the injury. Prognosis for recovery or adaptability can be similarly inferred.

Clinical neuropsychology grew out of years of research with persons who sustained brain injury, with the expectation that better understanding of the physiology of brain-behavior relationships could greatly assist treatment in many disciplines. Nurses, doctors, occupational and speech therapists, and other health care professionals use neuropsychological understanding in treating the whole person.

By application of a wide range of psychological tests and procedures, mental functions sensitive to brain injury can be measured objectively. Based on an analysis of the profile of scores and observation of the individual's problem solving processes, evaluation is made regarding (1) structural brain condition, (2) deficiencies caused by brain injury versus preexisting cognitive weaknesses, (3) strengths in cognitive and psychosocial skills, (4) comprehensive diagnostic understanding of the biopsychosocial impact of the injury, (5) extent of brain injury and prognosis for recovery, (6) the specific course of action needed for best therapy planning, and (7) predictions and recommendations for return to independence in work, school, and home.

Neuropsychological assessment usually starts very early during a person's rehabilitation. Even though a full neuropsychological assessment might not be appropriate or necessary early on, the neuropsychologist typically performs periodic testing of attention span, reaction time, short-term memory, and other foundations for higher cognitive functioning. As rehabilitation progresses and the individual improves, assessment becomes more comprehensive. Meanwhile, the neuropsychologist makes regular observations of the patient and interacts with him or her to gather impressions of how overall recovery is progressing.

A typical neuropsychological assessment involves undergoing several hours of tests, interview, and observation. The case history, including hospital records and laboratory tests, is reviewed in detail. The testing includes evaluation of attention span, concentration, orientation, memory, new learning, receptive and expressive language, mathematical reasoning, spatial perception, abstract and organizational thinking, problem solving, social judgment, motor abilities, sensory awareness, emotional characteristics, and general psychological adjustment. Tests are used as necessary to clarify diagnostic questions and make accurate predictions.

One of the key concepts in assessment of neurofunctional abilities is that of "executive functions." This refers to the individual's ability to think ahead, plan, pre-evaluate planned action, understand possible consequences, refine plans, take appropriate actions, and learn from successes and failures. Brain injury almost always affects executive functions to some extent. The neuropsychologist takes every opportunity to assess these functions and help the patient and treatment team know how to improve them or compensate for deficiencies.

Every person who has experienced a brain injury should have a comprehensive, formal neuropsychological assessment as soon as neurological stability has been reached. The neurologist, neurosurgeon, physiatrist, or brain trauma rehabilitation team can determine this stage when the patient slows down in rate of spontaneous neurological recovery, which typically will occur within a few months following injury. It is at this time that formal rehabilitative efforts, including occupational, speech, and cognitive therapy, are extremely important. Unfortunately, it is also at this time that lack of motivation begins to set in, as the person believes she or he is "back to normal" and does not understand the need for additional therapy. A neuropsychological assessment gives therapists the knowledge necessary to structure rehabilitation that will maximize continued improvement and minimize the effect of frustration on motivation when the patient cannot see functional improvement. Periodic (e.g., yearly) reevaluation by the neuropsychologist is necessary to record changes objectively and to monitor the effectiveness of treatment.

Other applications of the comprehensive neuropsychological assessment include its use as a patient and family educational tool, a treatment justification and plan for insurance carriers, a basis for educational or vocational rehabilitation planning, a basis for disability determination (for private insurance or for Social Security), and for life planning needs. By its nature, the neuropsychological assessment is comprehensive. It integrates the essential and unique diagnostic, prognostic, and treatment understanding about the individual.

Involving the neuropsychologist well before the first formal assessment is conducted provides an opportunity for interaction with the whole treatment team, the person, and the family. Assessing the extent and areas of brain injury thus can begin almost immediately after the injury occurs. By the time the individual is neurologically ready for a full evaluation, the neuropsychologist will have followed the course of recovery and will have made many behavioral observations. This will facilitate both drawing accurate inferences about the future course of recovery and defining therapy needs.

Once the person who has had a brain injury is physically and medically stable and a comprehensive neuropsychological assessment is completed, the major challenge of the next few years faces the individual and his or her family. Up to this point the course of action and care has been relatively routine and decisions have been made by the primary care physician. Now, without the need for acute hospitalization and constant attention to life-threatening conditions, or medical issues, determining the future course gradually is left more and more to the family. Usually, they are not well prepared to understand this new responsibility they face.

A comprehensive, detailed neuropsychological assessment, with periodic reassessments, can guide and assist the future course of rehabilitation, both in treatment facilities and at home. Neuropsychological consultations to supplement the assessment report provide realistic and scientifically based predictions of future recovery and the most potentially effective mixture of treatment and management approaches.

Armed with the detailed understanding of the neurological, cognitive, behavioral, psychological, and family dynamics that the neuropsychological assessment provides, the neuropsychologist usually becomes the primary care provider during the post-acute rehabilitation and later recovery stages. One of the most important roles of the neuropsychologist is to help families and the person who has had a brain injury make long-range decisions using the comprehensive information provided by the neuropsychological assessment.

This chapter identifies the critical components of a rehabilitation team and the team's major rehabilitation activities. The most common question asked by survivors is, "How long before I am recovered?" or the variant, "How long until I am normal again?" This is always a difficult question to answer because it is loaded with emotional consequences for the individual and family. Ultimately it is not readily answered with great precision. But, research has led to a better understanding of major predictors of recovery. Length of anterograde amnesia and findings of abnormalities on brain scans, for example, are significant indicators of severity of injury and expected recovery.

Anterograde amnesia is not the same as loss of consciousness. Anterograde amnesia refers to the recovery period when the person may be awake but not storing memory and subsequently is unable to recall that period of time. The period of loss of consciousness, alone, is not a reliable predictor of recovery, given the many factors that may contribute to a state of unconsciousness (such as use of sedation). Other factors play a major role in recovery, too, including age, years of education, pre-injury intellectual functioning, previous health problems, prior or current alcohol or substance abuse, a positive support network, previous employment, and access to rehabilitation and resources. The greatest rate of recovery is often between the three to six months post injury although other factors can be influential. The development of seizure, for example, can impact recovery in many ways.

Research suggests that much of the healing in the brain occurs within the first year following injury and neuropsychological test findings tend to be stable from that point forward. However, recent research indicates that recovery can occur for an additional 1-2 years, and points to the importance of ongoing diligence on the part of the individual in maximizing recovery through rehabilitation. Children and adolescents often have longer recovery periods because of the naturally active developing nature of their brain.

Concussion, or mild brain injury, is defined as a blow to the head that may cause no loss of consciousness or only a brief loss of consciousness— a period of altered awareness that typically leaves no findings on brain scans. During the conflict in Iraq and Afghanistan, the signature wound has been brain injury related to blast injuries (i.e., concussion). The after effects include sensory-motor and cognitive changes that may resolve within a few weeks. However, post-concussive headaches and other impairments may linger longer, sometimes much longer. The myriad effects of a concussion can include headaches, disrupted sleep, light sensitivity, and difficulty with attention and memory. Unfortunately, many individuals are sent home with the reassurance that they will be fine but with limited information on the likely recovery process and how they may facilitate recovery. Information about recovery is of substantial benefit to the individual in facing the challenges of a concussion. Medication to relieve headache and facilitate sleep may be helpful. A course of cognitive therapy can be fruitful in recovery and in return to job or school activities. Recent concussion care guidelines underscore the importance of managing the symptoms of concussion.

One of the most important challenges in brain injury recovery is to learn to retake control of one's life in a reasoned and realistic way. Rehabilitation is a necessary ingredient to recover optimal functioning and learn to advocate for oneself. Advocacy begins with an understanding of one's needs and then seeking out strategies, accommodations, and modifications toward reaching goals. In the process of rehabilitation, one learns what capabilities have been the most impacted by brain injury. One can then respond to this awareness by using effective strategies learned in rehabilitation.

The road to recovery typically begins with acute care. Once medically stable, the person moves to acute rehabilitation that requires more active participation in treatment. Many individuals hope and even expect that they should reach maximal recovery before being discharge from acute rehabilitation. This is far from typical. In the majority of situations, the individual is discharged from acute rehabilitation services within six months of the injury and given advice and direction on home-based programs, guidance on return to community participation (e.g., school, work), and available resources. Because formal rehabilitation is typically limited to a few hours a day or week (at best), self-advocacy is necessary for continuing to achieve maximum recovery. It is vitally important that an individual develops a plan and schedule to promote recovery and gradually increase participation in activities guided by information and support by one's family and health care and rehabilitation team.

Acute medical care is typically related to interventions to stabilize health. Rehabilitation, on the other hand, is interactive so that the key to success is the active involvement of the individual. Integration of one's environment, personal characteristics, capacity to participate with others, and bodily condition is necessary to achieve. This point has been reinforced at the pubic policy level by the World Health Organization's (2001) International Classification of Functioning, Disability and Health.

Rehabilitation must assess and intervene with each of these components. The rehabilitation team engages an individual through education regarding the changes that have occurred and the potential success through active involvement in rehabilitation. Rehabilitation engages the family and social network through education about changes associated with brain injury and teaches strategies and attitudes for promoting recovery. The critical role of a supportive and engaged family and personal support network cannot be understated in achieving positive outcomes. Rehabilitation must also aim to return the individual with a brain injury to life activities and social participation. Because a brain injury often results in some permanent changes, rehabilitation introduces the individual and the family to a road map for adapting to the changes. Adaptation often includes accepting and advocating for accommodations, modifications, and a willingness to see themselves or loved one in a different way.

Cognitive rehabilitation is forever. It begins with tasks that practice and enhance functional skills of attention, memory, reasoning, language, and related thinking skills. Simultaneously, the individual is beginning to learn and to use strategies for managing the changes in cognitive functions. In the long term, successful return to work, school, and home activities is largely related to the individual's development and consistent use of adaptive strategies. Cognitive rehabilitation should introduce an individual to ways that they can manage changes in cognitive skills, recognizing that doing so will enhance functioning in many areas of life. Naturally, time and experience help to refine strategies and typically reinforce their value.

Chapter Five

RECOVERY AND REHABILITATION

The challenge of brain injury first involves intensive, lifesaving medical and technical skill. The challenge then shifts to a focus on physical, educational or occupational, and neuropsychological restoration. The person with a brain injury and his or her family are better prepared for the long rehabilitation journey by understanding the stages of recovery and rehabilitation, the jobs of numerous therapists, and the many physical, cognitive, and psychological needs of the individual. The following sections offer this fundamental knowledge.

Primary Care

You are probably reading this book because you, a family member, or someone you know has sustained a brain injury. By now acute medical care has probably been provided. However, as a person remains under medical care and moves through the rehabilitation process, more health care professionals become involved. It is important in modern medical institutions that a primary health care professional be identified as the "primary care doctor." That individual takes charge of routing the patient through the maze of evaluations, treatment, management, and coordination of the other specialists. This individual also is the information provider, keeping everyone, including the family, informed of the patient's status and fielding discussions about the best options for optimum rehabilitation. Usually, this individual will change as the person with a brain injury either changes hospitals or facilities or becomes an outpatient. In any case, and at all times throughout rehabilitation, the person and his or her family need to seek the advocacy of the primary care doctor. These are usually the neurosurgeon, attending physician, physiatrist, or during later stages, the neuropsychologist.

Specialists within the Treatment Team

Modern medicine and rehabilitation is represented in an interdisciplinary team, not in a single person. The variety of specialists reflects the advancements and complexity of knowledge about brain injury, medicine, and rehabilitation, which cannot be the responsibility of just one or two persons. Integrated treatment requires the efforts of many professionals working together as a rehabilitation team. Among the variety of health care specialists, the following persons will likely be involved with the patient and family at some point:

Neurosurgeon: This individual is the key doctor and coordinator in emergency trauma treatment. He or she must have full control of the patient, being ready to intervene, with brain surgery if necessary, at any time. This doctor usually follows the patient through the acute phase.

Neurologist: After the emergency phase has past, evaluation of neurological status and medical management of brain disorder becomes the responsibility of the neurologist. Evaluation and reevaluations constantly monitor the patient's recovery. The neurologist frequently follows the patient beyond the hospitalization period, especially for seizure control.

Consulting Physicians: Depending on other injuries or circumstances unique to each patient, a variety of other physician specialists may be asked to consult, recommend, or treat. These may be specialists in pulmonary disease, orthopedics, cardiovascular problems, gastroenterology, or other areas.

Physiatrist: A physician specializing in physical medicine and rehabilitation often takes over primary care when the patient moves into a rehabilitation facility, but he or she may be called in to consult very early, particularly when other physical injuries are apparent. This physician usually directs and coordinates rehabilitation services in hospitals and is a specialist in the physical retraining of the body.

Neuropsychologist: Clinical evaluation of brain functions as reflected in behavior and emotions is the specialty of this psychologist. He or she may consult with other therapists and the family, and may conduct a variety of therapies to aid both the patient and the family with the psychological adjustment to trauma.

Rehabilitation Psychologist: Evaluation of and counseling for adjustment to the physical and mental changes brought about by brain injury is the special task of this psychologist, who understands the effects of bodily characteristics and change on mental state and attitude.

Rehabilitation Nurse: A nurse cares for the patient on a moment-by-moment basis and coordinates routine daily activities, including carrying out the doctor's medical management orders, attending to the patient's needs when the patient is unable to do so independently, and monitoring his or her physical and neurological health. This specialist is often the coordinator of several health and social services for the patient and family.

Social Worker: This professional is often the link between the patient/family and virtually all of the other care providers, as well as with the "outside world." The social worker may help resolve financial concerns, obtain rehabilitation equipment needed at home, provide emotional support for the family, and link the movement of the patient from facility to facility and eventually to home. The social worker is often the "case manager" who works with insurance carriers and community resources to assure smooth delivery of services.

Physical Therapist: This individual focuses on restoring physical use of the body to as high a level as possible. Teaching walking, posture, balance, endurance, strength, and coordination involves a complex program of skillfully designed exercises consistent with the physical and neurological potentials of the patient.

Occupational Therapist: Using the body to accomplish the familiar activities of daily living is the responsibility of the occupational therapist. Evaluation and treatment for regaining the use of fingers and hands, eye-hand coordination, self-care skills, eating, bathing, and learning numerous other functional skills requires knowledge and application of how the brain directs the body to carry out practical tasks.

Speech and Language Pathologist/Cognitive Therapist: Restoring language and thinking or intellectual skills is the specialty of the speech and language pathologist and cognitive therapist. Motor-speech, reading, hearing, and talking are retrained by involvement in graded programs, to strengthen conversational and other communication skills and to further develop higher level cognitive skills. These goals are geared toward re-integration of the patient into the family and community.

Recreation Therapist: Teaching the patient to make the most of leisure time, to enjoy relaxation, and to gain the necessary self-confidence for balancing work and play is the goal of this specialist. Patients often find themselves with much more time than they know what to do with, and the recreation therapist attempts to teach self-motivating skills so the patient can identify activities and use time satisfactorily. Music and art therapists also assist in restoring creativity, strengthening self-confidence, and encouraging healthy self-expression.

Respiratory Therapist: Patients experiencing breathing problems, particularly those on respirators, need assistance in adapting to such equipment to achieve proper oxygenation of the blood and in retraining the brain to once again carry out automatic breathing.

Psychiatrist: The physician who specializes in mental health is often called upon to evaluate problem behaviors and adjustment, particularly when medications can help. The psychiatrist is also a psychotherapist and may help the patient or the whole team in more effective behavioral management of the patient.

Nutritionist/Dietician: Proper diet is essential for maximum recovery of the brain and body. This specialist knows foods, nutrition, and proper weight control, and can also help patients and families develop good post-hospital diet plans. Patients who depend on gastric feeding are monitored for caloric and nutritional intake.

Vocational Rehabilitation Counselor: Once the person is sufficiently recovered from the acute phases of the trauma, this counselor may be of great benefit in helping clients make alternative employment plans. Often working in conjunction with cognitive rehabilitation professionals, the vocational rehabilitation counselor helps channel recovery into the directions essential for realistic plans for work re-entry.

Chaplain: The spiritual needs and desires of patients and their families are usually challenged in times of crisis. Helping families to accept what has happened and to make it through the uncertain times of early medical care tap the skills of the chaplain.

In truly interdisciplinary rehabilitation, all therapists share their specialty knowledge about a person with all other therapists. All team members, then, reinforce each other's work with the individual by assuring that all aspects of rehabilitation are always being applied no matter what individual therapist is working with the person at any given time.

As suggested earlier, following any disruption to normal body integrity, natural healing forces are activated. This spontaneous recovery begins very early and progresses for several months up to two years. Rehabilitation is the comprehensive and multifaceted process that channels the spontaneous recovery into efficient and maximum adaptability. Rehabilitation involves structuring the brain's relearning process to assist the individual in recovering as efficiently and as quickly as possible. It also involves learning new ways to compensate for abilities that have changed and may never be recovered as a result of the brain injury. The goal of rehabilitation is to recognize the unique characteristics of the affected person and to help him or her regain maximum independence.

Principles of Cognitive Remediation

By virtue of the nature of a brain injury, much of rehabilitation focuses on restoring mental, thinking, or intellectual functions. *Cognitive remediation* is the term applied to the activity characterizing this final (and lengthy) phase of brain injury rehabilitation. Though understood somewhat differently among therapists, cognitive remediation essentially helps the individual integrate thinking skills into the most effective and efficient use of brain resources. This involves learning memory improvement techniques, strategies for problem solving, methods for checking accuracy in arithmetic operations, concentration techniques, and other methods to improve cognitive skills. These procedures are reminiscent of school activities. Physical, occupational, speech, and other therapy specialists all eventually help the patient's brain direct all aspects of the body's and mind's functioning, and all are involved in cognitive remediation in some way.

A major focus of cognitive remediation, however, lies in psychological as opposed to educational concerns. It is common after a brain injury to develop some bad habits and attitudes that later interfere dramatically with independence. As the individual progresses through the recovery from a brain injury, two things occur that the family, particularly, must be aware of. Any acute care hospital setting may inadvertently teach dependency; by the nature of their structure, the ill person is "taken care of." Normally, people who experience a hospital stay do so for a relatively brief time. A person who has had a brain injury, however, may be in the acute care hospital for weeks or even months. During this same time, the brain is undergoing its most rapid recovery and is laying down new neurological connections producing behavioral patterns and habits. The kind of behavior the environment supports is the kind of behavior the brain will learn.

To help the patient move from the dependency and learned help-lessness that unavoidably begins in the acute care hospital, cognitive remediation must focus as early as possible on the individual's development of attitudes and beliefs that counteract the tendency to be dependent. Concurrently, as the brain reacts to its injuries, self- reflective thinking is not too abundant, yet self-conscious uncertainty is. Cognitive remediation, then, also focuses on encouraging the individual both to become aware of how he or she is thinking and behaving and to develop confidence in that thinking to carry out productive, intentional actions. Therapy also helps the individual to learn and practice efficient, independent, and appropriate behaviors.

A cognitive remediation therapy program aims to restore or to create functional systems. Such an effort proceeds in a sequence of activities as follows:

- Help the individual to recognize and accept the need for cognitive training based on his or her experience of changes or deficits. Enhancing awareness of problems and the need for help in resolving them make up the first step.

- Based on neuropsychological assessment, develop a set of realistic goals that will allow the individual to experience accomplishments and maximize independence in daily living.

- Design restorative training that is developmental, beginning with basic tasks and progressing to complex activities. Ample opportunity must be provided for task repetition, generalization, and practice of increasingly challenging skills. Training must be consistent and structured (predictable) for the patient. The neuropsychological assessment provides the foundation for determining the areas of need for training focus.

- Three specific areas of functioning that must be remediated are attentional, perceptual, and memory skills. These skills provide the foundation for all cognitive development. Thinking, organization, problem solving, and learning are all based on these fundamental skills.

- A monitoring system must provide frequent feedback to the individual on progress in basic functional skill development, relating these to broader goals for independence in living, education, or work. The difficulty level of these tasks must challenge the person but not overwhelm him or her.

Prognosis

Probably the single most reliable index of ultimate recovery is length of coma. The shorter the coma, generally the greater the recovery. Of course, there are other crucial factors, too, such as focal brain areas of damage, previous health history, the age of the individual, availability of therapy, specific nerve damage, bodily injuries, preexisting personality and coping resources, and rate of early recovery. As rehabilitation progresses, the rate of improvement serves as another index of recovery. The faster the improvement, usually the greater the ultimate recovery. However, recovery does slow down eventually. Although this may be disappointing, recovery can still be made for a long time, with the ultimate outcome unknown for months or years. Recovery takes much longer than most families expect.

Having some predictions for recovery is psychologically important; it helps reduce the anxiety of the unknown. However, neuroscientific knowledge is yet to be completely accurate in predicting recovery from brain injury. As discussed earlier, a person with a brain injury is never exactly as he or she was before the injury.

To deal with the unknowns in brain injury recovery, the best approach is one that assumes a dynamic, ever-changing brain. Persons with brain injury and their families must adopt the perspective that growth is always possible and available through hard work. Rehabilitation involves recovery and change. Continued use of educational and therapeutic resources, maintenance of realistic short-range goals, and the development of a positive emotional acceptance of "differentness" produces growth. This approach is applicable to anyone, brain-injured or not, for general life enrichment.

Just as ninety percent of cognitive remediation is psychological, most of rehabilitation generally lies in psychological attitude. Although we often epitomize "normality," it is being different, being proud, making the most of who we are and what we can do that gains respect and admiration. The challenge of rehabilitation is a new beginning.

Research shows that awareness of the changes and impact of injury occurs over the first 2 to 3 years. An individual with a brain injury well remembers life before the injury, and it should be no surprise that it takes time to understand what has and has not changed, and to integrate this into one's goals and activities. Attitude barriers to this process include catastrophizing, a spread effect, comparative thinking, and living in the past. Catastrophizing occurs when we think about a situation in the most negative light and as likely leading to catastrophic problems. The spread effect refers to expanding problems such that a person with memory challenges, for example, describes him- or herself as stupid. Living in the past occurs as a person returns to talking about him- or herself in the past, usually with the past being idealized. In comparative thinking, one tends to compare oneself with other groups, and usually in such a way as appearing now less functional or less fortunate. Each of these attitudinal barriers paints a negative picture and leads to a sense of hopelessness.

Learning adaptive coping attitudes typically involves cultivating a sense of hopefulness, positive problem solving, and flexibility. By this, we can come to a balanced assessment of our strengths and weaknesses, challenges and opportunities. When problems occur, we figure out ways around the block and come away with a sense of control in our lives. We appreciate that making mistakes is human yet we strive to not make the same mistakes and to learn from mistakes. We can appreciate that we may have to do things differently than we did them before. Adaptive coping is a lifestyle that we can recommend to everyone, whether a brain injury is involved or not.

Chapter Six

ACCEPTING AND COPING WITH CHANGE

The thought of long-term rehabilitation often bewilders families and the person who has had the brain injury. Implied are years of hard work, a long time before returning to pre-injury activity, and possibly physical or mental disability that is never fully recovered. The brain heals very slowly. But, the damaged brain can still learn, and, within limits, rehabilitation that is carefully planned and consistent with the physical condition of the brain and its intellectual strengths can produce positive and inspiring change. Good rehabilitation must be constantly monitored to assure that changes are progressing toward realistic goals.

In addition to an emphasis on recovery of functions, part of rehabilitation involves acceptance of permanent changes. People often have a difficult time with this, sometimes leading to denial or depression. An attitude that one must accept the things that cannot be changed, maintain the courage to change what can be, and grow to know the difference provides the balance that makes up rehabilitation.

Accepting and coping with change does not mean either "giving up" hope or "giving in" to a life of disability. Instead, acceptance and coping imply challenge, courage, and creativity. We have all too often heard people say, reluctantly, they guess they had better be happy with themselves and what they've got because there's always someone else worse off. This attitude suggests defeat and a feeling of self-resignation to some low status position even though they think they could be in even worse shape. This does not make one happy or challenged. Comparing oneself to others, better or worse off, is not psychologically healthy. Instead, adopting a prideful acceptance of who you are and a belief that you are so unique that you cannot rightly he compared with anyone else sets the stage for honest, self-respecting acceptance and coping.

This chapter explores some ways that family, friends, and the person with the brain injury can enhance acceptance of change.

Family and Friends

Early after a brain injury, while the person is in the hospital, in a rehabilitation center, or recently returned home, family and friends pay a great deal of attention. Friendly calls, cards, and gifts are a part of most peoples' recovery from an illness or accident. The nature of a brain injury may make it difficult early on to talk in much depth with the affected person or to see that they appreciate the visits and gifts. In fact, family and friends soon become aware that there is a child-like quality, even a childish self-centeredness, that characterizes the person. This often leads to gradually fewer and fewer visits. Friends may stop coming around or calling, and family members become perplexed, not knowing what to do or expect and feeling resentful about the abandonment.

It is vital to rehabilitation that the person with a brain injury learn about what has happened to his or her brain as soon as reasonable and become conscious of behaviors (impulsiveness, constant talking—especially about oneself, quick temper, etc.) that need changing. In addition, it is vital that family and friends learn that this individual's "problem" behavior is directly the result of brain injury. Although the person ultimately must learn to take control himself or herself, family and friends must learn to know what they can do to foster learning, adaptation, change, and eventual acceptance of those permanent residuals of brain injury.

Through love, understanding, and willingness to dedicate time to the family member or friend, positive growth does occur. There is, however, a point at which it must be recognized that the individual with a brain injury will not return to be exactly as he or she was before the accident. Thinking style may be changed, and social interaction will reflect that. Coming to terms with this is as much psychologically demanding for family and friends as it is for the person who has had the brain injury.

Guilt sometimes interferes with rehabilitation. Family and friends may feel uncomfortable when they reach the point of not knowing what to do next. If they abandon the individual, they may feel guilty; guilt usually leads to further withdrawal.

Fear of not knowing what to do or say or of not knowing how to react to unusual or unpredictable behaviors may contribute to destroying a relationship with the person who has had a brain injury. Fear of seizures or other physical or medical problems can be overcome through knowledge and forthright acknowledgment.

Uncertainty, confusion, resentment, guilt, pity—all of these emotions can characterize the family and friends of the person who has has a brain injury. These feelings neither help the person nor do much to foster understanding, supportive, or mutually satisfying relationships. Family consultation with the physiatrist, neuropsychologist, or other member of the rehabilitation team is beneficial, to keep everyone on track and to make the rehabilitation and adjustment process a positive one.

Some guidelines for relating to a person with a brain injury follow:

- Frequent but brief visits or phone calls are preferred over longer, infrequent visits.

- Being superficial destroys a relationship quickly. Be yourself; do not be afraid to ask questions; talk about yourself as much as you talk about the other person.

- Be informed about what has happened and seek education and understanding of what brain injury is all about.

- Talk over your feelings with someone if you are confused.

- Ask therapists who work with the individual how you can become involved in a helpful way in the evenings or on weekends when the therapist is not present.

The Person with a Brain injury

Family and friends best deal with accepting and adjusting to the changes brought about by brain injury, or any major life change for that matter, through a psychological process called "compartmentalization." Brain injury and its psychological impact is a part of people's lives only as they are around the person who has had the brain injury or are thinking of him or her. At other times, life can go on as before and not demand such intense adjustment. This is not so for the person with the brain injury; he or she is faced with the adjustment constantly. Certainly, this is not always unpleasant or even too demanding, but conscious awareness of how one is different or of what one needs to do to improve or adjust varies among people.

The major task for the person with a brain injury is to evolve a self-concept that integrates old and new characteristics, one that appreciates the need for self-respect and self-love despite differences that might be unfortunate and difficult to accept.

It is said that some of the most important aspects of rehabilitation begin long before the injury occurs. People who fear change, even disability, to the point of disdain will probably make poor rehabilitation clients. Someone who is rigid in thinking, who has a narrow acceptance of others and of right and wrong, who epitomizes normality, and who has few interests has not established a personality that can adapt to change very well at all. This is not to imply, however, that an injury cannot provide the impetus to make changes in one's attitude; indeed, it often does. It may just take longer.

Chapter Seven

MANAGEMENT GUIDELINES

Management may seem a harsh word to use in the context of the ideas presented in this book, but most persons with brain injury need some level of help and structuring throughout their lives. At first, this must be maximally provided by others, within a hospital or institutional setting. As rehabilitation progresses, though, it is expected that the person who has had a brain injury himself or herself can provide more of the day-to-day structuring to make life proceed smoothly. Reaching the balance between what one can do alone and what is needed from others is sometimes a battle of wits. Striving for independence is a strong goal, sometimes blinding one to the interfering effects of brain injury. Accepting realistically needed help while taking the challenges to increase independence (and sometimes to fail) requires sensitivity and trust.

Whereas the previous chapter focused more on the attitudes and values that lead to successful coping, the information that follows provides some specific guidelines for enhancing independence and quality of life.

Fundamental Principles for Family and Friends

A dozen general principles are offered here for family and friends, useful throughout the rehabilitation course. Each person is different and needs more or less help in specific areas. Managing the effects of brain injury is a joint venture (or, adventure) among the individual, family, friends, and therapists.

- Encourage rest or break periods either whenever frustration or fatigue appears or often enough to avoid their appearance. This will avoid discouragement or temper control problems.

- Keep activities and surroundings relatively simple. Too much, too fast, too soon leads to confusion and poor emotional control.

- Accept setbacks, both as a normal part of life and as a part of rehabilitation. Abundant encouragement and making light of setbacks assures overall growth. A sense of humor helps.

- Write things down that you want the person to do. Never expect that he or she will remember to carry out a sequence of tasks of more than one or two steps without this assistance. This assures the person of what is expected and that concrete rewards are given abundantly.

- Give honest feedback, with equal attention given to praise for desired behavior and brief, to-the-point, constructive criticism for undesirable behavior. Real sensitivity is required to achieve this balance.

- Surroundings should offer familiarity, predictability, and consistency, with regularly scheduled meals, activities, and rest.

- Do not surprise the person with a brain injury; explain activities fully before initiating them. Write things down, draw charts, use calendars, or whatever to serve as reminders of what is to come.

- Minimize confrontation or the use of logical argument for misbehavior. Redirecting the person's attention to something else is much more effective than either arguing or expecting the person to engage in a logical discussion.

- Being a model of calm, assured, confident behavior provides a sense of sureness and stability that the person wants and needs to build his or her own self-confidence. The person with a brain injury depends on others to re-learn how he or she should be acting or thinking.

- Providing specific choices from which to choose is more effective than requesting an open-ended, ambiguous decision. Persons with a brain injury can select from among things relatively easily, but they have unusual difficulty coming up with a decision spontaneously. (Left to a spontaneous decision, the choice may be quite inappropriate.)

- Use wall charts, reminder notes, labels, calendars, notebooks, journals, and other memory aids abundantly. Praise frequently when these are actually used by the person you are helping.

- Do not encourage challenge or competition which places the person with a brain injury at a considerable disadvantage with others. There is no need to increase either the chance of failure or the fear of failure, which leads to anxiety and defensiveness.

Tips for the Person with a Brain injury

A mutually cooperative attitude between the person with a brain injury and those close to him or her is certainly desired for optimum rehabilitation. Recovery is dependent on committed and persistent effort from everyone involved.

A group of individuals with brain injuries in a reintegration program, each at least two years post-injury, were asked to indicate one important "rule" they had to learn following their brain injury that contributed toward making life easier. Sixteen rules, or guidelines, emerged:

- Keep a detailed calendar of things you do and plan to do. This builds self-confidence, independence, and self-responsibility.

- Ask questions, but ask yourself first. Asking too many questions makes you dependent and not responsible for yourself and does not encourage your own critical thinking.

- Write things down. Keep lots of notes. This helps achieve multimodal learning; you hear it, write it, and see it. Just writing it down greatly helps you remember even if you don't ever look at your notes.

- Use no drugs or alcohol; these only dull the brain.

- Do not use mental delinquents like "I can't" or "oh, no." They remind us of negative thinking about ourselves. Be positive about what you can do.

- Do not use weasel words like "later," "maybe," or "kind of." These keep things vague and never commit you to anything.

- Keep a daily schedule. This establishes routines and helps make life predictable and easier.

- Have goals, but be realistic. Keep reassessing these goals to make sure you are actually achieving them and they are not just pipe dreams.

- Know yourself and what you can and cannot do. Be honest about this, and always make sure you are aware of what you are doing.

- Be on time.

- Always consider the optimistic side of things.

- Be willing to do new things. Don't just "try." Do!

- Be outgoing to get along with others; accept others; do not judge others; respect individuality.

- Be organized.

- Do not be the center of attention.

- Do not be afraid to accept help.

Chapter Eight

RESOURCES

When the person with a brain injury leaves the acute care hospital, the myriad rehabilitation services sometimes overwhelm families. Knowing what resources are available for what purposes allows a family to know they are not alone, that there are others "out there" who are ready to help. The course of treatment following acute care varies with the needs of the individual. The acute care treatment team will assist families in planning the stages of rehabilitation and the selection of facilities. Unfortunately, what facilities and services call themselves versus what they actually do is sometimes confusing. The following information is offered to help sort out that confusion.

Depending on one's physical needs, it is usually valuable to continue work in physical and occupational therapy beyond that provided in the acute care hospital. This will facilitate the return of fine and gross motor coordination. Although one's rate of improvement may slow considerably over a few months post-injury, increments in coordination capability may still be experienced as the brain continues its slow healing process. Continuing these efforts will pay off in increasing potential for independence and opportunities for return to work.

Speech and language therapy is an important aspect of rehabilitation in that brain injury almost always disrupts communication skills, even in very subtle ways. Depending on the individual's specific treatment needs, therapy usually focuses on speech production (rate, volume, articulation, etc.), organization of thinking, language comprehension, reasoning skills, and other language-related areas.

Cognitive remediation involves focused training in thinking and reasoning skills, including organization of thoughts and time, using calendars and other aids for time and self-management, planning activities and goals, sequencing to follow through on tasks, problem-solving and decision-making strategies, improving mental speed and flexibility, and mathematical reasoning such as money management and budgeting. Many agencies offer such training, often through specially trained speech therapists.

Psychotherapy is beneficial for many individuals who have sustained a brain injury and their families as they struggle with how the experience has changed their lives and influenced their interaction with others, at home, school, job. and social gatherings. Family members also often need a period of assistance in accepting change, learning to develop or accept realistic expectations, developing strategies for assisting their family member to improve or manage specific behaviors, and in being supportive of their efforts. The behaviors of the person must be understood in light of his or her physiological damage and not as merely learned maladjustments.

Various forms of medical attention may be necessary to assure seizure control or the maintenance of special physiological conditions brought about by the brain injury. Such resources are available through a private neurologist, physiatrist, or other physician who is familiar with brain injury.

Educational and vocational rehabilitation assistance may be needed for continuing education and job training or retraining. State and private rehabilitation agencies offer such services. A checklist is provided in the following section to review for possible contacts or other resources.

Emotional Support

The topic of emotional support is singled out for special attention. Families need to avail themselves of informational and support groups usually offered through an affiliate the Brain Injury Association of America, through local rehabilitation facilities, or through local community colleges or other organizations.

State Brain Injury Associations can be contacted for a wealth of information on local, state, and national rehabilitation programs and facilities, financial and legal advice, educational materials and programs, family support activities, Social Security disability and insurance benefits, recreational and social support activities, and other areas of interest or concern. Most organizations welcome volunteers to help with their programs. Volunteering is a great way to get to know and learn from others, and to feel good about yourself by helping others.

Families and persons with brain injury almost always, sooner or later, seek the mutual support and understanding various organizations offer. Going through any emotionally demanding experience is lonely. Having others to encourage strength and to explore the challenge with is important in maintaining mental health.

A Checklist of Resources

Have these people or agencies been considered? (All resources may not available in some areas)

- Brain Injury Association of America — *www.biausa.org*
- Local or state associations of the BIA America, such as Brain Injury Association of Kansas sand Greater Kansas City — *www.biaks.org*
- State Department of Vocational Rehabilitation (or private vocational agencies)
- Special programs for persons with brain injury or learning disability offered through adult education or community colleges
- Special education coordinators
- Local family support groups
- Rehabilitation agencies and hospitals for outpatient support programs and/or therapies
- Local parks and recreational agencies that have programs for special groups
- Local volunteer placement
- Agencies and organizations providing home and community based services
- Schools and community colleges
- Transitional Living programs
- County extension offices

Types of Rehabilitation Facilities

The array of rehabilitation facilities and programs can be intimidating or at least confusing. There is only a weak standard for labels, and what a program calls itself may not be what one thinks it is. The labels provided below identify several major categories of programs and facilities, from acute care to independent living. Programs are often not mutually exclusive, and the services they offer may overlap. These descriptions are only a guide; it is up to the individual and the family to investigate a specific program to determine its suitability. Here, again, the experience of others can be useful in meeting unique needs.

Acute Care Rehabilitation. Within the acute care medical facility, a designated rehabilitation unit might exist. Patients are moved into that unit, or to such a unit in another medical center, as soon as they are medically stable. Similar intensive rehabilitation is sometimes provided in a specially designated facility which itself does not have an attached medical or emergency trauma unit. The primary emphasis of acute rehabilitation is to provide intensive physical, occupational, recreational/educational, psychological, and speech therapy in the early weeks after injury or after coma resolution. Most such facilities will have specialized traumatic brain injury sections with a comprehensive interdisciplinary team. These inpatient programs are of relatively short duration, usually lasting a couple of months, but longer if necessary.

Post-acute Rehabilitation. When a person no longer needs the intensity of acute care rehabilitation, a milestone of independence has been reached. Post-acute rehabilitation may be just as intense as acute care rehabilitation. However, the person usually no longer needs the day-to-day care of the rehabilitation nurse, and is safe to spend nights and weekends without so much, or any, direct supervision. Treatment intensity focuses on cognitive remediation and educational or vocational re-entry.

Long-term Rehabilitation. Facilities that are able to provide longer-term rehabilitation often provide a more residential-like, as opposed to hospital-like, setting. Such a program is necessary for the patient who is making slow improvements and needs longer-term intensive therapy and support services. Such facilities generally are not considered for permanent placement, but a person may remain in the program as long as some improvement continues to be demonstrated.

Special Problem Programs. Many residential or inpatient rehabilitation programs are designed for specific emphasis in aspects of
trauma rehabilitation. This might be coma management, an experi-
mental program in limb control, an intensive effort in cognitive and
socialization retraining, a behavior management program, an occupational reentry program, or a nursing home program specifically designated for brain injury treatment. There are many such programs,
and overlap exists among them. Sometimes programs are referred to
as "subacute" or "skilled" facilities for those with medical problems,
and "post-acute" facilities for those needing continued therapy but
minimal medical attention.

Extended Rehabilitation Facility. The more seriously injured person
may require extended, intensive, and comprehensive therapies in a
structured program, having elements of several special problem programs as well as the acute rehabilitation center. Cognitive retraining,
speech therapy, memory retraining, skills of daily living, restructur-
ing lost social behaviors, and continued physical therapy characterize such programs. Prevocational and vocational training, recreational
therapy, and community reentry are usually part of the program. Resi-
dents may remain in the program as long as progress is being made.

Transitional Rehabilitation. The main goal of a transitional program
is to prepare individuals for maximum independence, to teach skills
useful in community interaction, and to work on vocational goals, if
appropriate. These programs are similar to extended or post-acute rehabilitation facilities, but take the form of small group homes or special programs within educational institutions. Their goal is to provide
the steps necessary to achieve independent living.

Residential Living. For those individuals unable to live at home or
otherwise to live independently, a structured group residential facility
may provide the appropriate placement. Very few facilities of this type
exist specifically for people with brain injuries, but growing concern
for their need may change this situation in a few years.

Nonresidential Reintegration Programs. Day treatment services
are created to upgrade functional skills, including usual physical and
occupational therapies, cognitive therapy, psychosocial adjustment,
prevocational training, independent living skills, and so on. Such
programs are community based and may be offered through private

agencies, hospitals, or colleges. They are similar to the post-acute or transitional programs.

Respite Programs. Short-term "vacation-like" opportunities are being recognized as important for patient and family to get away from each other for a while. Like residential living facilities, these are not plentiful, but such programs are recognized more and more as crucial in the long-term rehabilitation challenge, especially for the more seriously injured person.

Financial Resources

One of the most difficult and frustrating aspects of brain injury rehabilitation is cost. Facilities and professionals' time are expensive. Considering the intensity and extent of need, the cost of rehabilitation of a person with a brain injury, aside from the primary acute medical care, can run into hundreds of thousands of dollars. A comprehensive medical insurance policy is invaluable, but even that is no guarantee that it will cover all of the person's needs. Whatever the resources available, insurance, personal finances, or accident settlement, it is important to seek the assistance of a trusted financial advisor. State affliates of the Brain Injury Associasion of America usually can be of invaluable assistance in these matters.

Legal advice is often necessary to help clarify responsibilities for covering medical and rehabilitation costs, securing disability benefits, obtaining protective guardianship arrangements, and pursuing personal injury claims. Educational programs relative to these needs are periodically provided by support agencies.

Anyone who has to sort through the resources for brain injury rehabilitation will quickly recognize and appreciate the presence of new friends—those who have gone through it before. Severe brain injury often changes virtually every aspect of a family's life. Medical, physical, psychological, financial, spiritual, emotional, and social challenges face everyone whose life is touched by brain injury. Challenge is measured by one's ability to accept reality, to give tirelessly, to adapt to change, to direct hostile energy into creative activities, and to love. To live life anew, to experience the joy of triumph, to have faith in life itself—these are the ingredients of happiness for anyone. We hope the information in this book helps increase knowledge and foster insight that provides the basis for successful coping.

GLOSSARIES

Hospital Equipment

arterial line: a catheter placed in an artery, used to monitor blood pressure in the arteries and to allow for access to arterial blood for laboratory studies.

catheter: a hollow tube placed into a part of the body for the removal of fluids or to allow fluids to be introduced into the body.

central venous pressure (CVP) line: a catheter that is threaded into the right atrium of the heart. The CVP reading directly reflects the right ventricular filling and diastolic pressure in the right atrium of the heart.

chest tubes: tubes that are placed into the chest to drain fluid from the body.

endotrachial tube: a tube that is inserted into the trachea through either the mouth or nose to ensure an open airway.

Foley catheter: a catheter that has a small inflatable balloon on the end, usually inserted into the bladder. The balloon is inflated to keep the catheter in the bladder so that urine can be continuously drained into an external bag.

halo: a metal ring used with patients who have spinal cord injuries to preserve proper alignment of the neck and spinal columns. This helps keep the patient still and the body aligned during healing.

intracranial pressure monitor: a monitor, inserted through the skull, that measures pressure of the fluid inside the brain and skull.

intravenous (IV) line: a small catheter placed into a vein, which can be used to give a patient fluids, drugs, or blood; also used to monitor venous blood pressure.

intravenous board: a board that is used to hold an extremity immobile so as not to dislodge an IV line.

monitor: any machine that gives a reading of vital body processes, such as cardiac (heart) monitors or intracranial pressure monitors.

nasogastric tube: a tube inserted through the nose into the stomach, through which to feed a patient, to give medications, etc.; used if a patient is unconscious, has severe jaw injury, or is unable to swallow.

respirator/ventilator: machines that either assist a patient with breathing or actually breathe for him or her by forcing oxygen into the lungs.

space boots: large, soft protective shoes used to support muscles and tendons during coma.

Swan-Ganz catheter: a catheter that is threaded into the heart and wedged in a pulmonary arteriole; used to measure pulmonary artery pressure and pulmonary capillary wedge pressure, both good indicators of left ventricular function.

traction: traction devices apply a pulling force to reduce, align, and immobilize fractures; to lessen, prevent, or correct deformity associated with bone injury and muscle disease; and to reduce muscle spasms in fracture of a long bone or in back injury.

transducer: a device that changes input energy of one form into output energy of another. For example, physiological energy such as the heart beating is changed from beats to lines on a strip of paper that can be read.

ventriculostomy: an operation that is performed to drain fluid from a ventricle of the brain to treat hydrocephalus.

Medications

The following is a sample of medications used in caring for persons with brain injury. New medications are regularly introduced that may not appear in this list.

antibiotics: a category of medications used to control the infections to which injured persons are prone.

Baclofen: relieves muscle spasms and muscle tone problems.

BuSpar: used to alleviate anxiety.

Dantrim: relieves muscle spasms, cramping, and tightness of muscles.

Decadron: a cortiosteroid used to reduce inflammation and improve brain functioning through reduction of brain swelling.

Dilantin: used to control or prevent seizures and convulsive disorders.

Haldol: used to calm agitated, combative, anxious, or tense patients, usually during the relatively early stages of post-acute treatment.

imipramine: used as an antidepressant.

Lasix: used to reduce excess water from the body and help reduce intracranial pressure, water in the lungs, or sluggish kidneys.

laxatives: a category of drugs used to encourage bowel movements and to relieve constipation.

Maalox: used to help prevent stomach ulcers or stomach discomforts that hospitalized patients are prone to develop.

Mannitol: removes water from the brain, used to decrease intracranial pressure.

morphine sulfate: used to reduce pain and to reduce bodily reflexes through sedation.

Mysoline: an antiseizure medication, often used if other similar-acting drugs fail to work.

Nembutal: used to reduce intracranial pressure and reduce pain.

Pavulon: used to relax skeletal muscles to help keep the patient from struggling, usually while on a respirator.

phenobarbital: used to control or prevent seizures and convulsive disorders.

Prozac: used as an antidepressant.

Ritalin: used as a brain stern stimulant to help improve attention and concentration.

sleeping medications: a category of drugs used to assist in maintaining regular sleep/wake cycles; examples are Dalmane, Halcion, Restoril.

steroids: a category of drugs used to reduce brain swelling.

Tagamet: used to help prevent stomach ulcers to which hospitalized patients are prone.

Tegretol: antiseizure medication that also effects impulsive behaviors.

Valium: used to reduce anxiety, tension, and muscle activity.

Xanax: antianxiety medication to help reduce tension and muscle activity.

Neurological Tests and Procedures

BEAM (brain electrical activity mapping): a computerized analysis of background EEG activity, much more sensitive than conventional EEG, which is especially helpful in identifying abnormalities of early dementia or suspected brain injury from brain injury.

brain stem evoked responses: brain stem response to a specific stimulus recorded electronically.

CT scan (Computerized Tomography): computerized x-ray taken at different levels of the brain to yield a three-dimensional representation of the physical shape of the brain.

electrocardiogram (ECG or EKG): electrical measure of heart activity and heartbeat that is produced on a chart recording.

electroencephalogram (EEG): an evaluation of electrical activity of the brain.

lumbar puncture: a tap into the spinal fluid to assess presence of toxic agents or infections that might be present in the brain.

MRI scan (Magnetic Resonance Imaging): an instrument that develops images from biochemical operations of the brain by using a magnetic field.

neurological examination: an assessment of gross nerve functioning via reflexes and reactions; performed by a neurologist or neurosurgeon.

PET scan (Positron Emission Tomography): an instrument that records chemical activity in specific regions of the brain.

Neuropsychological Terms

abstract reasoning: process of generalizing from concrete examples and experiences to larger, broader principles.

acalculia: dysfunction or inability to perform mathematical operations, recognize numbers, or count.

acuity: keenness of sensation.

agnosia: loss of ability to recognize familiar people, places, and objects.

agraphia: loss of ability to express thoughts in writing. alexia: inability to read or recognize words.

anomia: dysfunction or inability to name objects or recall individual names.

anterograde amnesia: loss of memory for events and periods of time following an injury or traumatic event.

apathy: decrease in motivation, initiation, interest in life and growth; indifference.

aphasia: loss in ability to speak coherent ideas or understand spoken language.

apraxia: loss of ability to carry out habitual movement or acts that were previously automatic.

astereognosis: inability to recognize objects or shapes by feeling them.

asymmetry: discrepancy in function or appearance between sides of organs.

ataxia: dysfunction in motor coordination and balance.

attention: ability for sustaining focus on task for a period of time to allow for coding and storing of information in memory.

cognition: processes of thinking, understanding, and reasoning.

concentration: ability to remain attentive to a specific task for a sufficient time.

diplopia: seeing two superimposed images of a single object; "double vision."

disinhibition: loss of restraint or decrease in ability to stop oneself from saying or doing something that is typically undesirable.

disorientation: disturbance in recognition of person, place, and/or time and day.

dysarthria: disruption or dysfunction in speech articulation.

emotional lability: intense fluctuations of emotions in response to experiences.

frustration tolerance: amount and degree of frustration; encounter with obstacles one can live with before losing control over affect and thinking.

inflexibility: rigidity in thinking; over reliance on stereotypes; difficulty in recognizing alternative possibilities.

judgment: ability for resolving dilemmas and approaching problems; includes values, morals, and interpretation with respect for interactions.

memory: stored recollections about experiences, events, feelings, dates, etc., from the recent and distant past.

perseveration: over-reliance on or repetition of a specific response or behavior to different tasks.

post-traumatic amnesia: loss in memory for events related to a traumatic event and the period immediately following the trauma.

problem-solving: skills for employing reasoning, judgment, experience, and discernment in resolving problems.

retrograde amnesia: loss of memory for events and periods of time before an injury or accident.

unilateral neglect: unawareness or inattention to one side of the body or the space or events occurring on one side of the body.

visual field deficit: inability to perceive vision in an area of the visual field, such as the right or left field, known as hemianopsia.

APPENDICES

Glasgow Coma Scale

The patient is rated on the following scale in each of the areas indicated: eye opening, best motor response, and verbal response. The scale is used during the initial assessment after injury and for monitoring recovery during coma emergence. A score of 3 indicates deep coma while a score of 15 indicates no coma at all.

Eye Opening (E)
opens eyes spontaneously	4
opens eyes when asked loudly	3
opens eyes to pain (pinch)	2
does not open eyes	1

Best Motor Response (M)
obeys simple commands	6
localizes motor response	5
withdraws body part to pain (pinch)	4
flexes body inappropriately to pain (decorticate posturing)	3
body becomes extended in response to pain (decerebrate)	2
no motor response at all	1

Verbal Response (V)
normal orientation and conversation	5
confused and disoriented in conversation	4
articulates but uses inappropriate words that make no sense	3
incomprehensible sounds only; no conversation	2
makes no sounds	1

The total Glasgow Coma Scale score is the sum of the E, M, and V ratings. Minimum score is 3; maximum is 15.

Revised Rancho Los Amigos Scale

The revised ten-level Los Amigos Rancho Scale takes up where the Glasgow Scale leaves off. The Rancho is more appropriate for judging where a person is in terms of overall recovery from a brain injury. The scale covers a long range of time, from coma to maximum recovery. It is based on the generally observed sequence of recovery characteristics of the typical person with a brain injury. Since no one follows a sterotyped pattern, the Scale provides only a general sense of where the individual is in terms of brain healing. Individual characteristics must be taken into account.

Level I, No Response: No response to pain, touch, sound, or sight. Completely unresponsive.

Level II, Generalized Response: Generalized (gross), inconsistent, non-specific reflex response to stimuli (usually pain). Responses usually delayed.

Level III, Localized Response: Specific but inconsistent response to stimuli such as blinks to strong light, turns toward/away from sound, responds to physical discomfort. Inconsistent, delayed response to commands. Vague awareness. May show some response bias toward some persons.

Level IV, Confused-Agitated: Alert, very active, aggressive, inappropriate, confused behaviors. Performs motor activities but behavior is nonpurposeful. Extremely short attention span, lacks recall, gross attention to environment. Detached from present and responds primarily to own internal confusion. Poor discrimination.

Level V, Confused, Inappropriate, Non-agitated: Appears alert but only gross attention to environment, highly distractible, requires continual redirection and structure. Difficulty learning new tasks. Agitated by too much stimulation. May engage in social conversation but with inappropriate verbalizations. Self-care behaviors usually performed.

Level VI, Confused-Appropriate: Inconsistent orientation to time and place. Retention span and recent memory impaired. Begins to recall past and show some learning carryover. Consistently follows simple directions. Goal-directed behavior with assistance. Begins to show awareness, recognition but selective attention still somewhat impaired.

Level VII, Automatic-Appropriate: Performs daily routine in highly familiar environment in a non-confused but automatic robot-like manner but dependent on some external direction. Skills noticeably deteriorate in unfamiliar environment. Lacks realistic planning for own future. Judgment and problem-solving impaired for realistic self-appraisal.

Level VIII, Purposeful-Appropriate: Alert, oriented, able to recall past and recent events, responsive to culture. Independent. Shows carryover and can learn activities. Vocational rehabilitation appropriate. Some lingering judgment difficulties.

Level IX, Purposeful-Appropriate with Stand-by Assistance on Request: Able to perform and complete tasks. Aware of impairments and able to compensate by corrective action. Able to self-monitor appropriate behavior with stand-by assistance.

Level X, Purposeful-Appropriate Modified Independent: Able to handle multiple tasks simultaneously. Independently initiates steps to complete tasks but may require compensatory strategies to complete. Appropriate awareness of impairments and how they may impact activities of daily living. Social interaction behavior is consistent.

ABOUT THE AUTHORS

Dennis Swiercinsky, PhD, ABN

Dr. Swiercinsky began his neuroscience career as director of neuro-psychology at the Topeka Veterans Administration Hospital in 1975. He transitioned to private practice in Kansas City in 1980 and has since worked primarily with clients who have sustained a brain injury. Dr. Swiercinsky served on the board of directors for Brain Injury Association of Kansas and Greater Kansas City. He headed the Neuro-behavioral Unit at Laguna Honda Hospital in San Francisco for two years and now practices criminal forensics in Portland, Oregon. His book, *Normal Again: Redefining Life With Brain Injury,* reflects his nearly 30 years in diagnostics and treatment of persons with traumatic brain injury.

Terrie Price, PhD, ABPP

Dr. Price is the Director of Neuropsychology and Family Services of The Rehabilitation Institute of Kansas City. Her previous work has included working alongside co-authors, Dr. Swiercinsky and Dr. Leaf, in private practice. She has served on the boards of professional organizations, including Brain Injury Association of Kansas and Greater Kansas City and Brain Injury Association of Missouri. She was a contributing author of *The Missouri Greenbook: Living with Brain Injury* (2009), distributed by Missouri Department of Health and Senior Services. In collaboration with state colleagues, she contributed to a training curriculum for educators in Missouri for returning kids to school following brain injury. She was on an expert panel to the CDC on surveillance of head injury in children.

Leif E. Leaf, PhD

Dr. Leaf was formally the Neuropsychologist/Clinical Director for a neuro-rehabilitation program in Las Vegas. Dr. Leaf is a nationally recognized expert and conference speaker on topics related to neuropsychology, behavioral management and traumatic brain injury. As a former speech language pathologist, Dr. Leaf's interests include working with adults and children with anxiety-related disorders, family issues, and organic brain syndromes. Dr. Leaf is currently in private practice in Kansas. He has served on the board of directors for Brain Injury Association of Kansas and Greater Kansas City.

ABOUT BIAKS

The Brain Injury Association of Kansas and Greater Kansas City (BIAKS) is a not-for-profit organization comprised of people with brain injuries, family members, friends, and professionals. BIAKS is part of a network of brain injury associations across the United States, and is a chartered affiliate of Brain Injury Association of America. We are the only organization in Kansas serving individuals with brain injury, their families, and the professionals who treat them. We are dedicated to providing information, advocacy, and support to those we serve.

BIAKS relies on the generosity of others for meeting our programming needs. Donations can be made through our secure website, *www.biaks.org*. Donations for any amount are greatly appreciated.

Ordering Information

Additional copies of Traumatic Head Injury: Cause, Consequence and Challenge are available for purchase. Ordering information can be found on our website, www.biaks.org. All proceeds from the sale of these books go directly to BIAKS to help meet programming needs.

On behalf of the staff and board of directors of BIAKS,
we thank you for your continued support.

50529910R00049

Made in the USA
Charleston, SC
29 December 2015